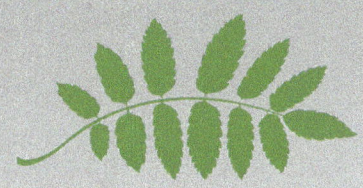

WEST END ORGANIX

Ageless Beauty, Organic Health

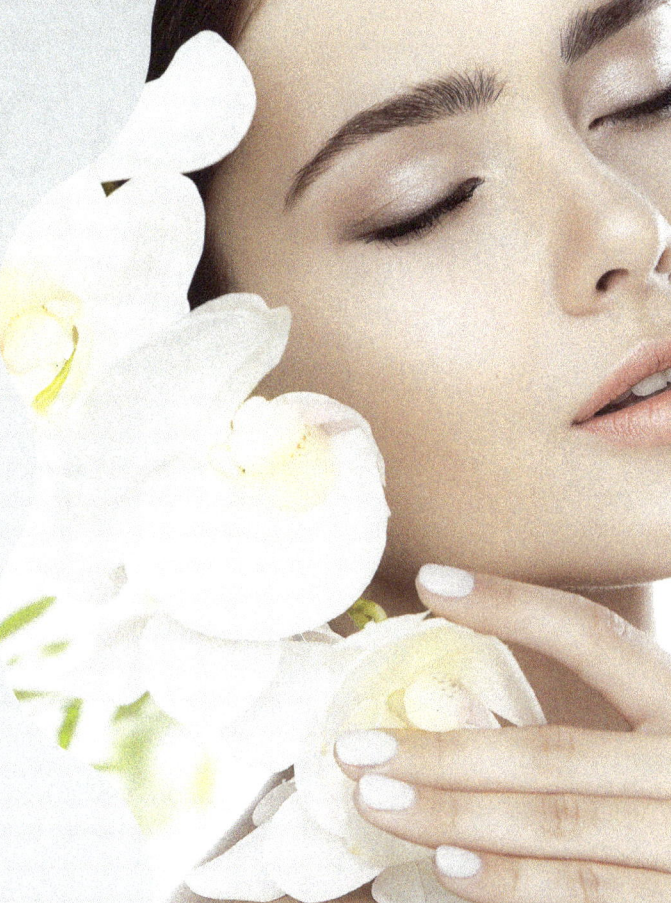

Look and feel younger and healthier with our natural remedies products!

www.WestEndOrganix.com

Discount: 10% off of your order - Code *WEO2021*

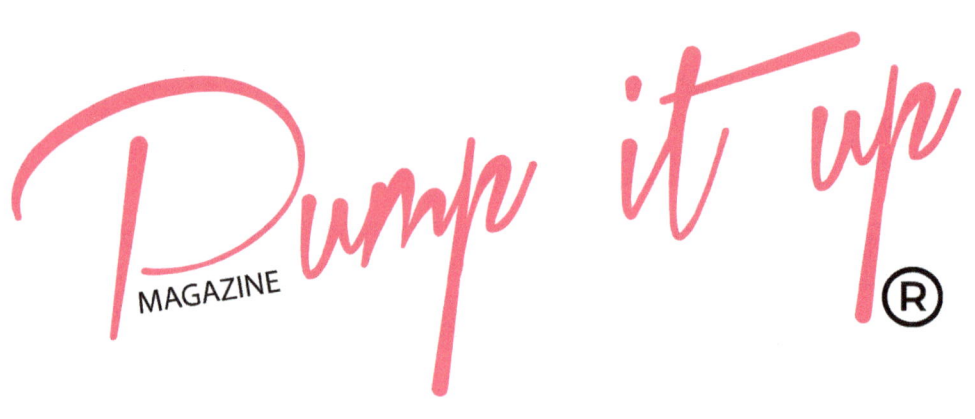

Pump it up

MAGAZINE ®

PUMP IT UP MAGAZINE ———

LINKS

WEBSITE
www.pumpitupmagazine.com

FACEBOOK
www.facebook.com/pumpitupmagazine

TWITTER
www.twitter.com/pumpitupmag

SOUNDCLOUD
www.soundcloud.com/pumpitupmagazine

INSTAGRAM
pumpitupmagazine

PINTEREST
www.pinterest.com/pumpitupmagazine

PUMP IT UP MAGAZINE
30721 Russell Ranch Road
Suite 140
Westlake Village,
California 91362
United States

 (818)514 – 0038(Ext:102)

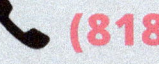 **info@pumpitupmagazine.com**

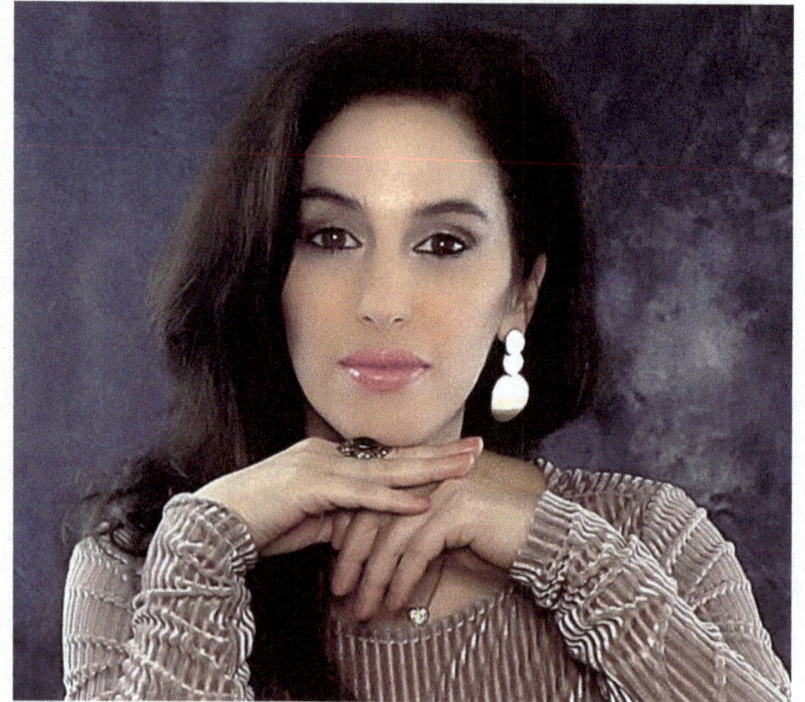

Greeting Readers!

We're thrilled to announce that Ingram Street
is this month's cover star on Pump it up magazine
! You need to know about Minquel and Woody,
a popular R&B duo, if you want to be hip to the latest music!

Pump it up magazine will cover different great topics
to prepare you for an amazing new year!
Find out how to look like a celebrity in our fashion section.

There will be no more excuses for not getting fit in 2023! You'll w
to check out our fitness feature!

You'll find all about natural ways to fight wrinkles on the beaut
pages.

If you're thinking about traveling in a motor home,
our article will tell you the pros and cons of it.

Our learn French feature will help you get ready
if you're planning a trip to Paris.

We've got a great selection of music for your road trip vacation
Our movie section also features some of the best Oscar-worthy
films of the year.

We will also share some strategies for getting your music heard
more people in our top tips section!
Finally, in our humanitarian awareness section, you will learn
how to help stop human trafficking.

Happy New Year!

Anissa Sutton

CONTRIBUTORS

EDITOR IN CHIEF
Anissa Sutton

MUSIC
Michael B. Sutton

MARKETING
Grace Rose

PARTNERS

Editions L.A.
www.editions-la.com

The Sound Of L.A.
www.thesoundofla.com

Info Music
www.infomusic.fr

Delit Face
www.DelitFace.com

L.A. Unlimited
www.launlimitedinc.com

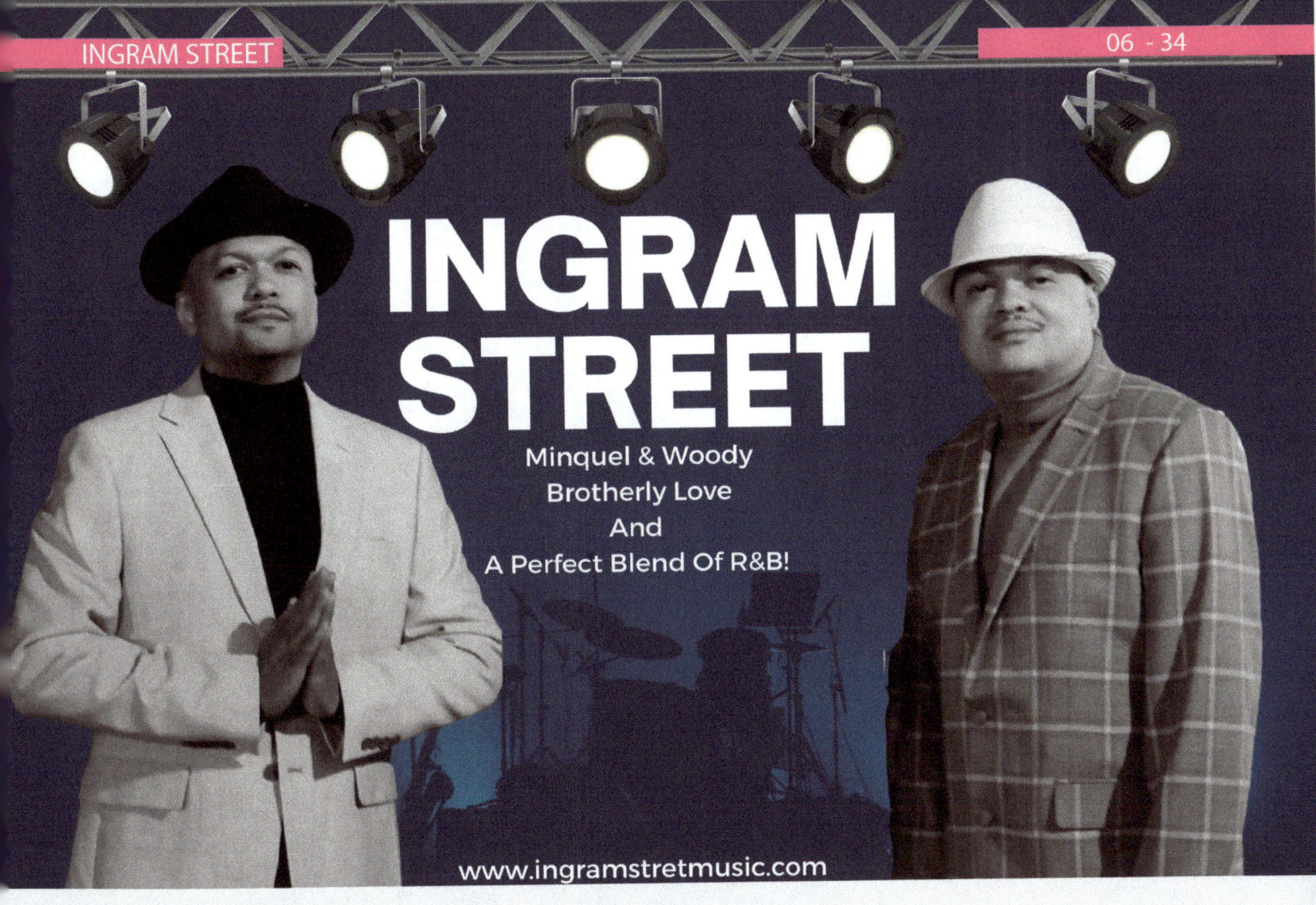

INGRAM STREET

Minquel & Woody
Brotherly Love
And
A Perfect Blend Of R&B!

www.ingramstretmusic.com

For as long as a decade now, INGRAM STREET has put a smile on our faces each time with its outstanding sound of Rhythm and Blues (R&B). Especially since much of R&B music is widely associated with the natural feeling of Love, their newest single "Natural High"(The Realm Remix) does not fall far from the euphoric feeling.

Exemplifying the trademark of their sound, the single "Natural High"(The Realm Remix) comes off with a laid-back soul vibe that will get you attracted to its melody. Its true love theme is an exhibition of the natural forces of attraction between two people that are completely and entirely attracted to each other.
The single comes through as the first number off their forthcoming remix album "Streetlights" which is anticipated to release in April this year (2023).

INGRAM STREET as a music duo have been doing music since they were in Grade school. Already with two studio albums in their bag; "Escapism" & "Paint The Town" and several singles, they have continuously proved their ingenuity in music and largely within the genre of R&B. Some of their earlier musical influences were the likes of; Mr Phillip Ingram, Maxwell, Debarge, and The Jacksons.

Following closely in familiar footsteps, the duo has steadily grown their discography into a likeable work of art and have been able to achieve this by surrounding themselves with positivity and only people that believe in what they do.
Their newest single "Natural High"(The Realm Remix) is the latest display of their undisputed talent and will surely hit as hard when you turn it up on that date night, Anniversary, or even on an ordinary day with your loved ones.

Head to INGRAMSTREETMUSIC.COM all major music streaming platforms, including Spotify to listen to "Natural High"(The Realm Remix) by Ingram Street.

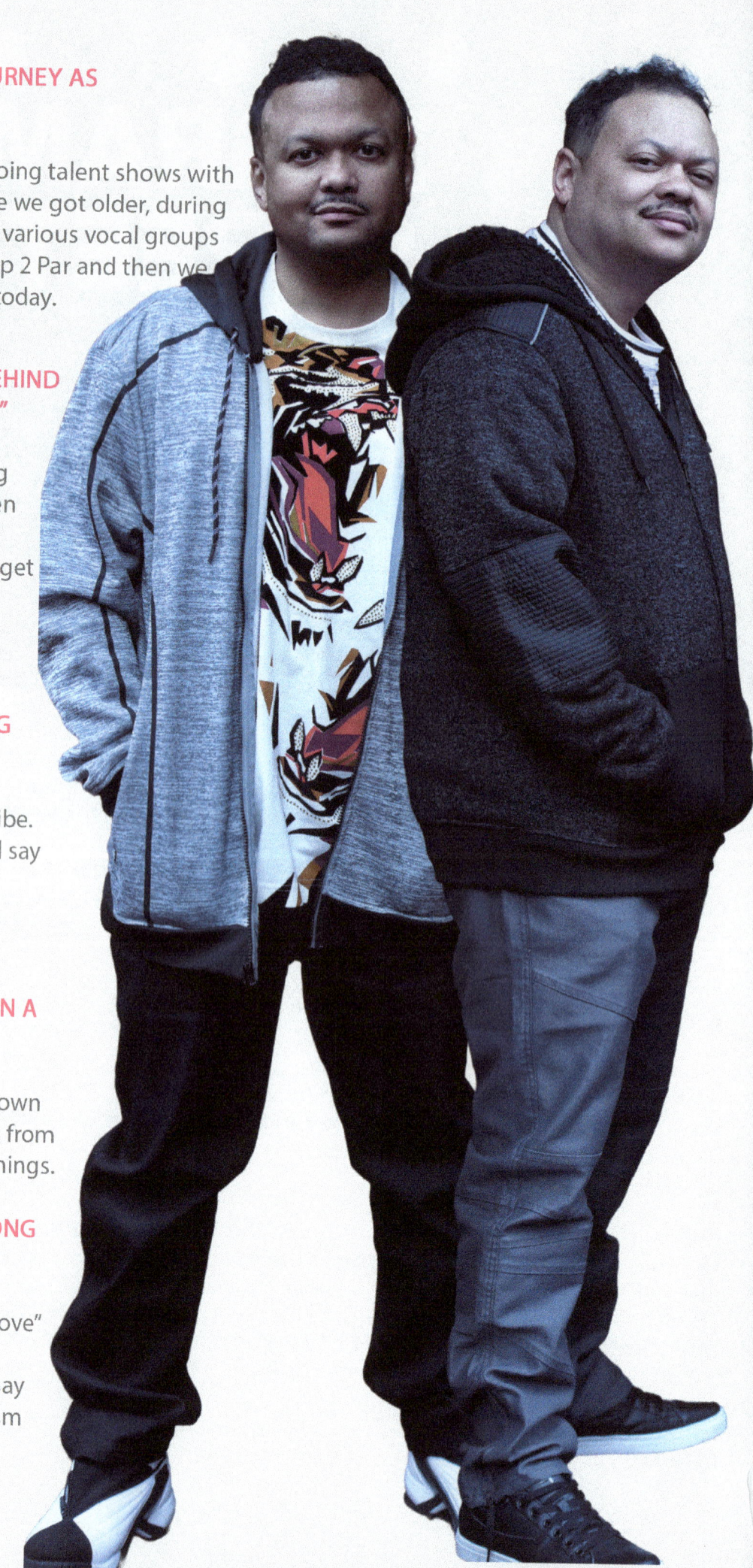

1. TELL US ABOUT YOUR JOURNEY AS INGRAM STREET?

We got started really young doing talent shows with our sisters for our family. Once we got older, during out teenage years, we formed various vocal groups including Combination and Up 2 Par and then we downsized to the duo we are today.

2. WHAT IS THE MEANING BEHIND YOUR SONG "NATURAL HIGH"

Natural High is a true love song about the feeling you get when you are with someone You are attracted to and the vibes you get when your around them just being in their presence.

3. WHAT ARE THE MUSICAL INFLUENCES FOR YOUR SONG "NATURAL HIGH?"

The song has a laid back soul vibe. Some of the influences, I would say are Maxwell, Debarge, and The Jacksons.

4. HOW DO YOU DIVIDE THE RESPONSIBILITIES OF BEING IN A BAND?

Since we are a duo, we split it down the middle, pretty much 50/50, from artistic to the business side of things.

5. WHAT IS YOUR FAVORITE SONG YOU HAVE WRITTEN?

Minquel "Don't Disturb This Groove" From our Escapism album.
Woody: for me I would have to say "Euphoria" also from our Escapism album.

6. HOW DO YOU FEEL WHEN YOU PERFORM IN FRONT OF A LIVE AUDIENCE?

The energy I feel is amazing, it is almost euphoric and I love connecting in person with the audience through the music.

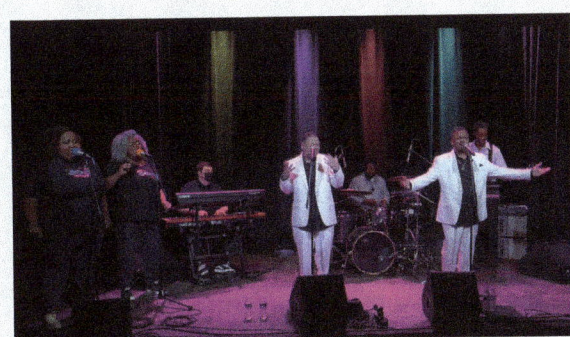 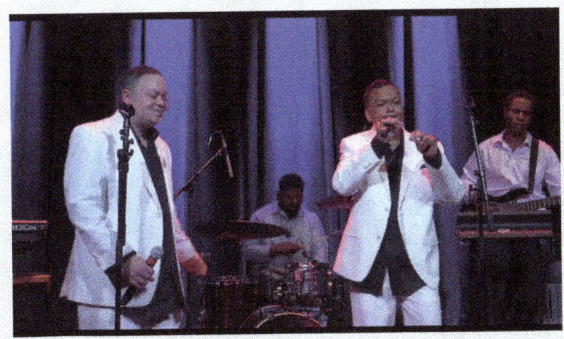

7. WHAT WAS YOUR MOST MEMORABL MOMENT AS A BAND?

Being able to do a virtual concert with one of our musical influences, Mr. Phillip Ingram.

8. WHAT IS YOUR FAVORITE SONG BY ANOTHER ARTIST?

Minquel: Too many to name, but if I had to go with one, I would say "Wildflower" by New Birth Because it reminds me of my mom.
Woody: I agree there are so many.
I will say "Sweet November" by The Deele, I have always wanted to write a song like that.

9. WHAT WAS THE FIRST SONG YOU EVER WROTE AND HOW DOES IT COMPARE TO YOUR NEW SINGLE?

The first song we ever wrote together where we got a positive response was a song Called "I Saw You In My Dreams" Our mom lit up when she heard us sing it. We were in Grade school when we wrote it so we didn't have the life experience we have now, but It was a ballad, just like "Natural High."

10. WHAT IS THE PROCESS FOR YOU WHEN COMING UP WITH MUSIC TOGETHER?

Early on, we would come up with the lyrics and melody first and then have someone Put the music to what we came up with; however, we mostly receive tracks from Various producers and we will put the words and melody to the track if it speaks to us.

11. WHAT IS THE BEST ADVICE YOU HAVE EVER RECEIVED FROM SOMEONE ELSE ABOUT ACHIEVING YOUR GOALS?

Surround yourself with people who believe in what you are doing and support you.

12. WHAT'S NEXT FOR INGRAM STREET?

Our new remix album "Streetlights" which will include "Natural High." It should be out in April. More shows and an EP release of all new songs by year end.

INGRAM STREET

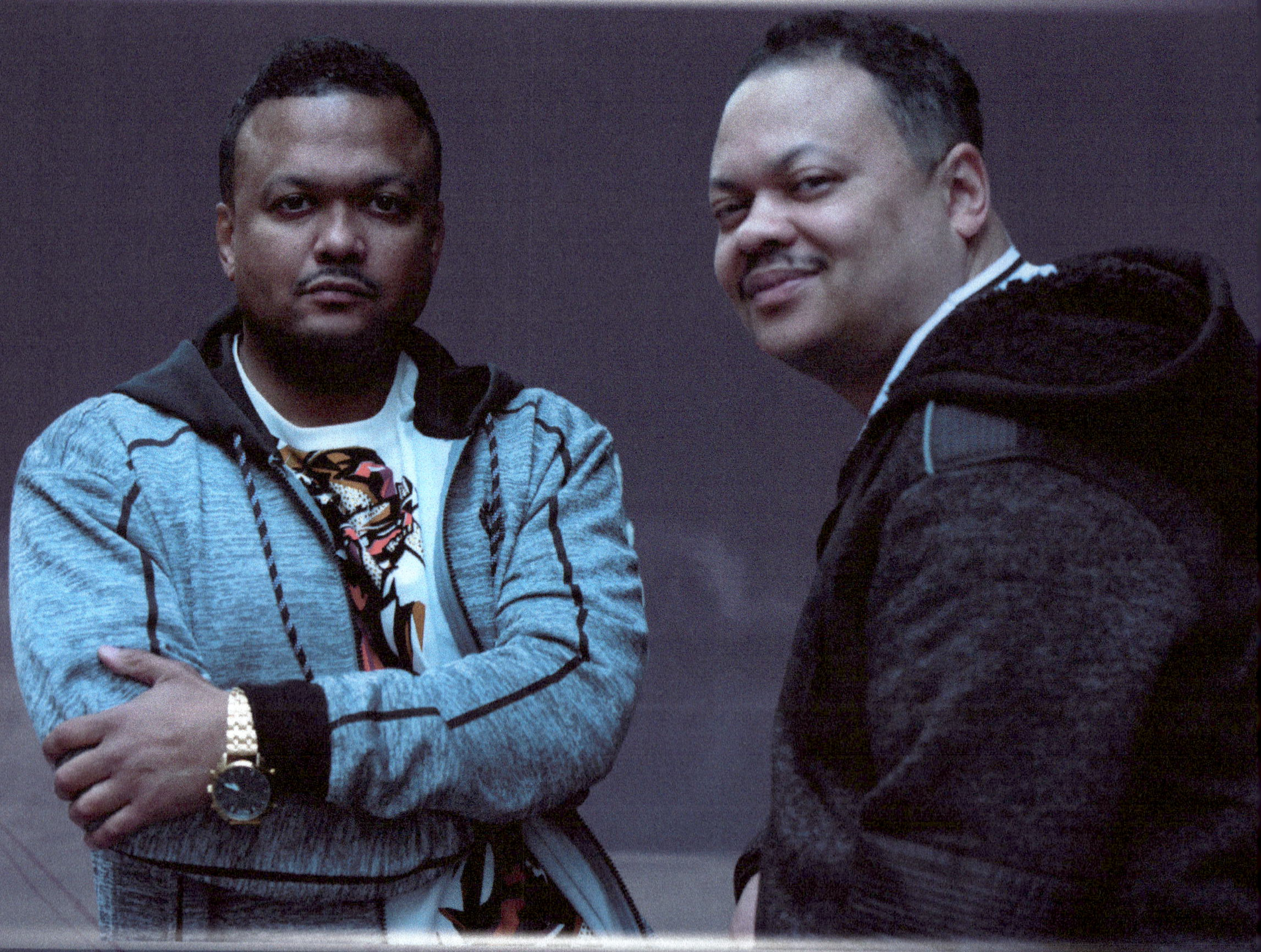

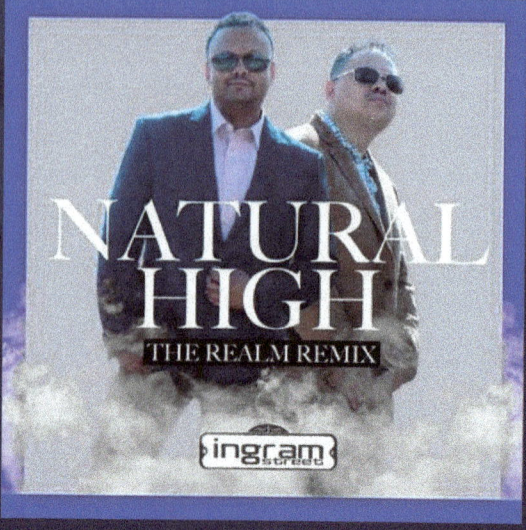

presents

THEIR NEWEST R&B REMIX!
"NATURAL HIGH" (THE REAL REMIX)
ONE YOU DON'T WANT TO MISS!
SO GET READY TO TURN UP THE VOLUME AND EXPERIENCE A
NATURAL HIGH WITH INGRAM STREET!

AVAILABLE NOW: WWW.INGRAMSTREETMUSIC.COM

WHY TRAVEL IN A MOTOR HOME?
THE PROS OUTWEIGHTS THE CONS!

When it comes to travel, there are a lot of options to choose from.
You can go by plane, train, bus, or car.
But have you ever considered traveling in a motor home?
Here are some of the pros of doing so:

WHY TRAVEL IN A MOTOR HOME?

There are many reasons to travel in a motor home. Perhaps the most important reason is that it allows you to have your own home with you wherever you go. This means that you can cook your own food, sleep in your own bed, and relax in your own living room. It also means that you can save money on hotels, since you can simply camp out in your motor home instead.

Another reason to travel in a motor home is that it is a great way to see the world. You can travel to any destination that you want, and you can do it at your own pace. You also have the freedom to explore different parts of the world without having to worry about where you will sleep or eat each night.

Finally, travelling in a motor home is a great way to meet new people. You will have the opportunity to meet other travellers who are also exploring the world, and you will also have the chance to meet locals who can show you around their hometowns. This can be a great way to learn more about a new place and to make some lifelong friends.

THE PROS OF MOTOR HOME TRAVEL

There are many benefits to motor home travel.
For one, you have your own private space where you can relax and feel at home.

There is no need to worry about noisy or disruptive passengers, and you can come and go as you please. Additionally, you have all the amenities of home with you on the road, so you never have to go without your favourite comfort foods or drinks, or feel like you're missing out on your favourite TV shows.

Motor home travel is also a great way to see the country or world at your own pace, and to explore destinations that may be off the beaten path.

THE CONS OF MOTOR HOME TRAVEL

There are several disadvantages to traveling in a motor home.
For one, they can be very expensive to operate.

Gas prices can really add up, and you'll also have to pay for campsites or parking fees.

Additionally, they can be difficult to maneuver, and can be a hassle to drive in city traffic.

Finally, they can be quite cramped, especially if you're traveling with a large group.

EXPLORE
The World

WHY YOU SHOULD CONSIDER TRAVELING IN A MOTOR HOME

Freedom

When you travel with a motor home, you have the ultimate freedom to explore the world. You can go wherever you want, when you want and stay as long as you desire. No need to worry about finding a place to stay, looking for public transportation or dealing with airline tickets!

Affordability

You'll save money on accommodation since you'll be staying in your own self-contained living space. You'll also save money on food costs since you'll have a fully functioning kitchen in your motor home. Not to mention, you'll save money on transport as your motor home will get you from point A to point B.

Comfort

You will have access to a full kitchen, living area, sleeping quarters and bathroom, all in one vehicle. This means that you won't have to worry about packing up your things each time you move from one place to another. Plus, you don't have to worry about expensive hotel bills when you stay on the road for long periods of time.

BOOK NOW

123981 Craftsman Rd., Calabasas, CA 91302

1(818) 225-8239

www.expeditionmotorhomes.com/

GET READY FOR YOUR NEXT TRIP TO PARIS
LEARN FRENCH TODAY!

So you're thinking of taking a trip to the most romantic city in the world – Paris?
If you want to be able to communicate with the locals,
you'll need to know some basic French phrases.
Here are a few to get you started.

LEARN THE BASICS OF THE FRENCH LANGUAGE.

In order to learn the basics of the French language, one must first understand its structure. French is a Romance language that derived from Vulgar Latin. It is considered to be one of the most difficult languages to learn for English speakers. The French language has several unique features that make it difficult to learn, such as its verb conjugation and its use of nasal sounds. However, with a little bit of effort, anyone can learn to speak and understand basic French phrases.

STUDY COMMON PHRASES AND VOCABULARY.

In order to improve your language skills, it is important to study common phrases and vocabulary. This will help you to understand and be understood by others. There are many different ways to learn new words and expressions. You can use a dictionary, a textbook, or an online learning resource. You can also listen to native speakers and try to imitate their pronunciation.
If you are looking for an easy way to learn French, "How to start a french conversation in french" is for you! It is easy to follow and you will learn the basics of the language. This will help you have a conversation in French while on your trip to Paris

PRACTICE YOUR CONVERSATIONAL SKILLS.

You know how important it is to be able to hold a conversation in a foreign language. But even if you're comfortable with the grammar and vocabulary, you might still feel a little shy when it comes to actually speaking the language. Here are a few tips to help you get over that hump and start speaking like a pro.
1. Find a conversation partner. The best way to improve your conversation skills is to practice with a real person. Find someone who is also learning the language, or someone who is a native speaker. You can meet people online or in person, depending on what works best for you.
2. Use flashcards. If you're not comfortable meeting people face-to-face, you can always use flashcards to practice. Just make sure to actually say the words out loud, not just read them in your head.
3. Watch movies and TV shows in the language you're learning. Not only will this help you improve your comprehension skills, but you'll also get to hear how native speakers actually speak the language.
4. Don't be afraid to make mistakes. Everyone makes mistakes when they're learning a new language. The important thing is to not be afraid to make them and keep trying.
With these tips, you'll be well on your way to becoming a conversation champion.

YOUR TRIP TO PARIS

Paris is one of the most popular tourist destinations in the world, and with good reason. There is so much to see and do in the City of Lights.
From the Eiffel Tower to the Louvre Museum, from Notre Dame to the Arc de Triomphe, there is something for everyone in Paris. And of course, no visit to Paris is complete without a visit to the infamous Moulin Rouge!

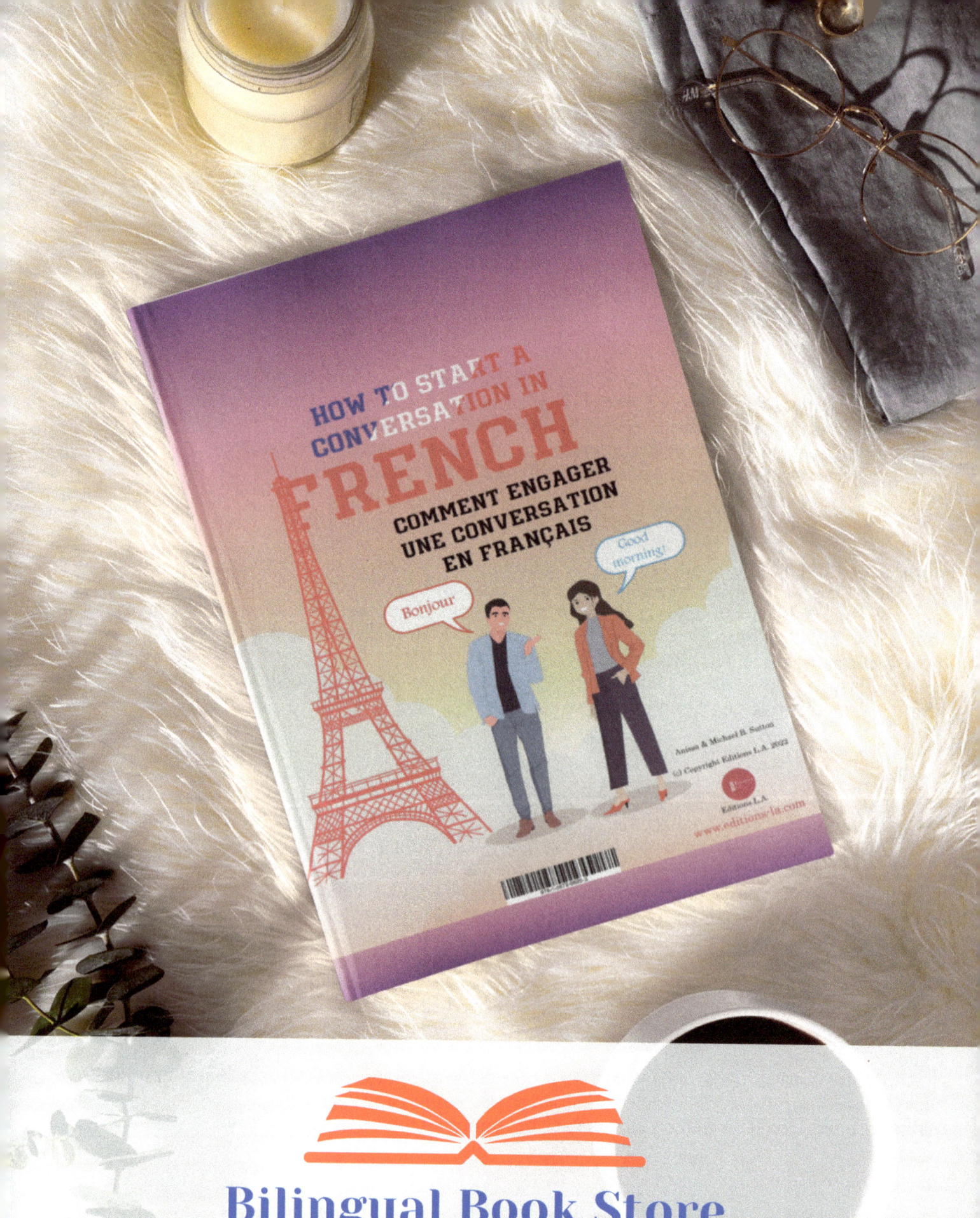

THE BEST ROAD TRIP MUSIC FOR YOUR NEXT VACATION

No matter what your road trip music preference is, there is surely a playlist out there to fit your needs. Whether you want to listen to the latest pop hits or old school rock favorites, there's something for everyone.
So, what are you waiting for? Start packing for your next vacation and get ready to sing along to your favorite tunes!

INTRODUCING SOME OF THE BEST ROAD TRIP MUSIC FOR YOUR NEXT VACATION.

Whether you're driving through the countryside or stuck in traffic on the interstate, these tunes will keep you entertained and help you stay relaxed and focused on the road. So pull out your headphones and get ready for a musical journey.

1. "Life is a Highway" by Tom Cochrane
This classic road trip song is perfect for getting your journey started on the right note. It's upbeat and positive, and its lyrics will help you to enjoy the experience of hitting the open road.

2. "Take It Easy" by The Eagles
This mellow song is the perfect soundtrack for cruising down the highway on a sunny day. It's easy to listen to and will help you to relax and take things easy while you're on the road.

3. "I'm on a Road to Nowhere" by Kenny Chesney. This song is a great choice if you're looking for a more mellow road trip song. It's a bit slower and more relaxing.

4. "California Dreamin'" by The Mamas and the Papas
If you're headed to the west coast, you'll want to add this classic song to your road trip playlist. It's the perfect tune to listen to as you drive through the California landscape.

5. "Walking on Sunshine" by Katrina and the Waves
This upbeat song is perfect for driving down the highway with the windows down. It

TIPS FOR MAKING THE MOST OF YOUR ROAD TRIP MUSIC.

Road trips are a lot of fun, but they can also be long and tedious. That's why it's important to make the most of your road trip music. Here are some tips for doing just that:
1. Make a playlist ahead of time.
If you have a specific list of songs that you want to listen to, it'll be a lot easier to keep the trip moving. Plus, you can always customize the playlist as you go.
2. Plan your route around your music.
If you're traveling to a new destination, try to plan your route so that you can listen to your favorite songs while you're driving. This will make the trip feel a lot shorter.
3. Sing along!
Not only is singing along with your favorite songs a lot of fun, but it can also help you stay awake on long road trips.
4. Bring headphones.
This one is a no-brainer. If you want to listen to your music without disturbing anyone else, bring some headphones.
5. Take advantage of free music streaming services.
There are a lot of great free music streaming services out there, like Spotify and Pandora. So if you're looking for some new tunes to listen to on your road trip, be sure to check them out.

★★★ — ANEESSA
MICHAEL B. SUTTON

I FOUND MYSELF IN YOU

OUT NOW

WWW.THESOUNDOFLA.COM

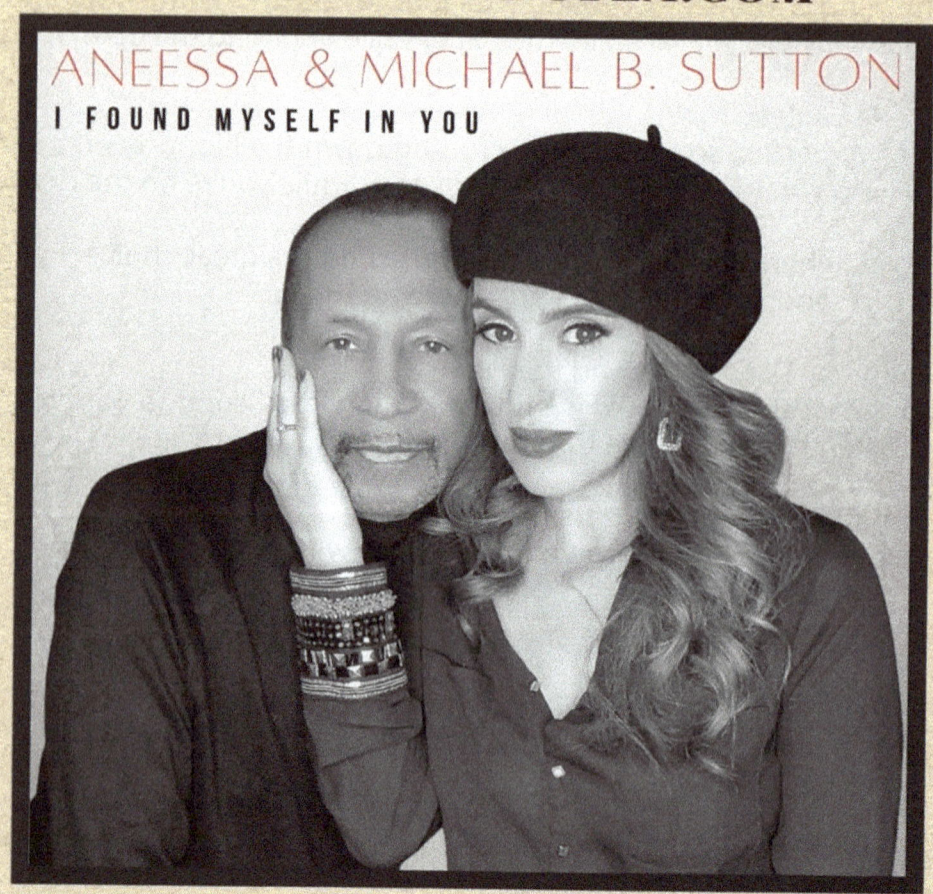

   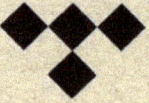 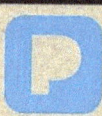 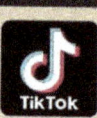

*Smooth Jazz Love Song
for An Essential Romantic Playlist
Capturing the joyful essence of
what it feels like
to love and be loved!*

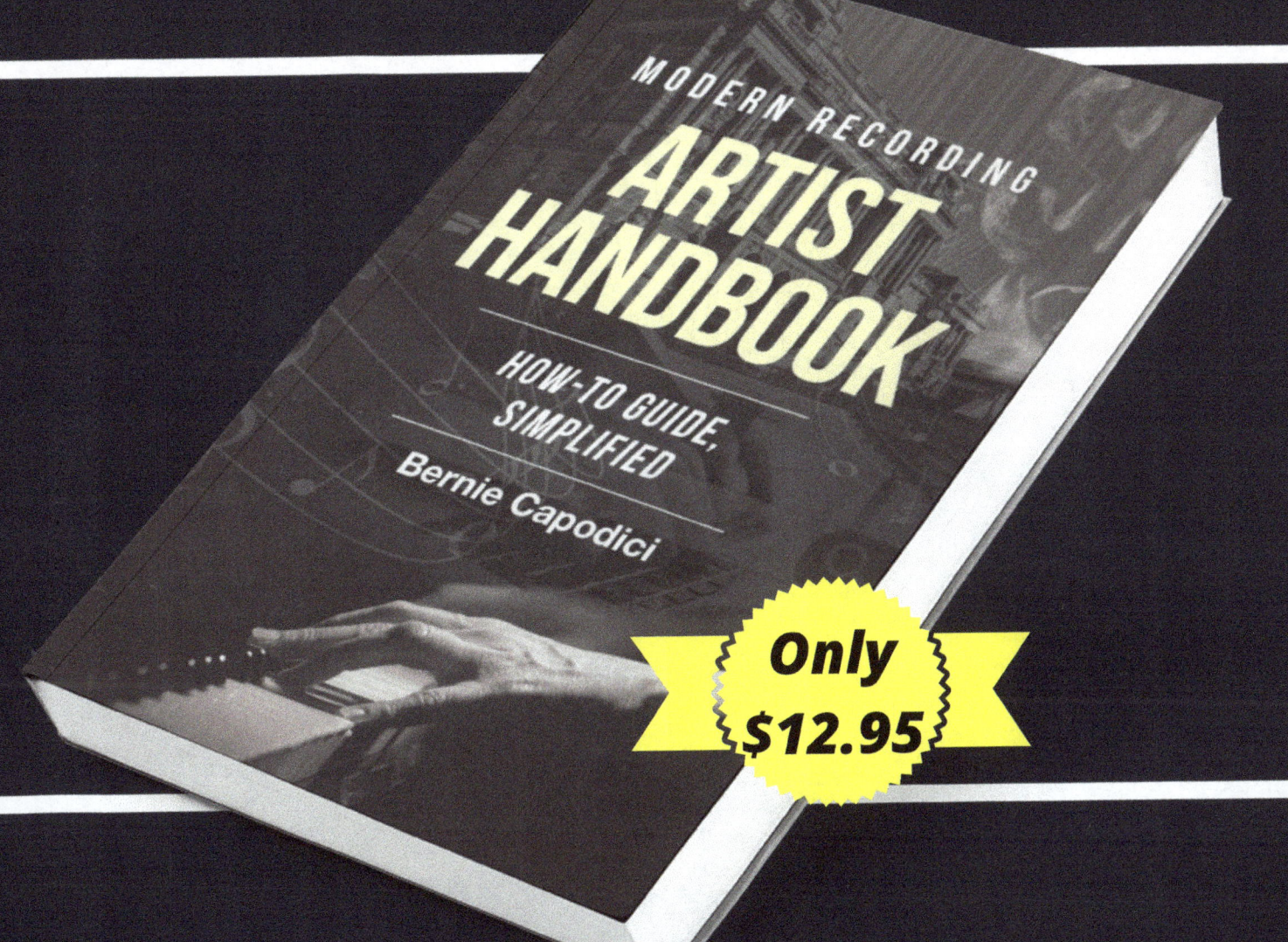

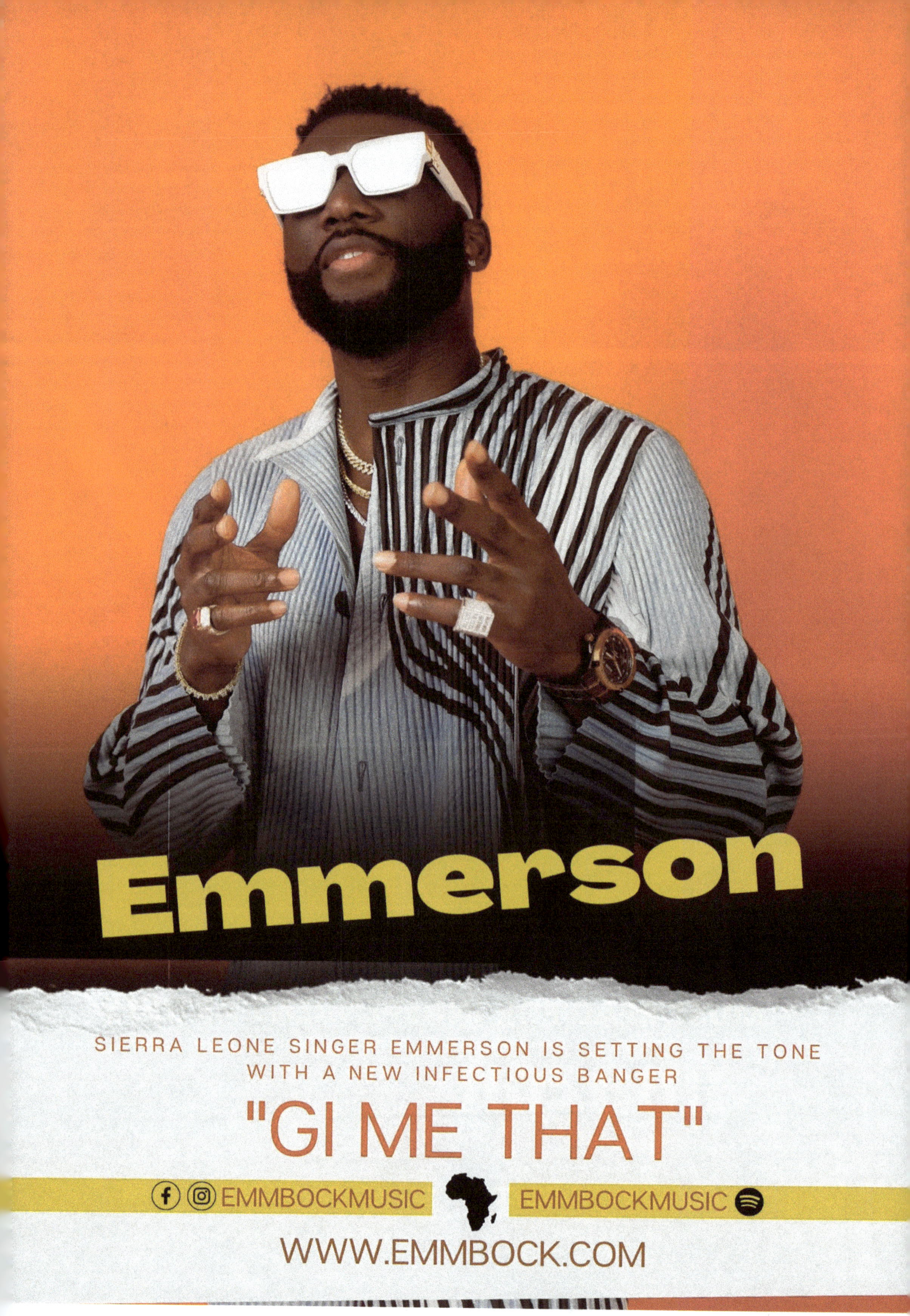

Emmerson

SIERRA LEONE SINGER EMMERSON IS SETTING THE TONE
WITH A NEW INFECTIOUS BANGER

"GI ME THAT"

 @EMMBOCKMUSIC EMMBOCKMUSIC

WWW.EMMBOCK.COM

HOW TO LOOK LIKE A STAR: NEW YEAR, NEW LOOK!

If you're looking to start the new year with a new look, you're in luck!
There are plenty of simple tips and tricks you can use to make yourself look like a star.
Keep reading for some helpful ideas.

DRESSING FOR YOUR BODY TYPE

When you're looking for the perfect outfit, it's important to think about your body type. Dressing for your body type can help you look your best and feel more confident.
If you're apple-shaped, you'll want to wear clothes that create the illusion of a smaller waist. Try wearing dark colors on the bottom and lighter colors on top. You can also wear tops with details on the waist, like a belt or a wrap.
If you're pear-shaped, you'll want to wear clothes that draw attention to your upper body. Try wearing darker colors on the bottom and lighter colors on top. You can also wear tops with details on the waist, like a belt or a wrap.
If you're hourglass-shaped, you'll want to wear clothes that show off your curves. Try wearing clothes that fit your body well and show off your curves. You can also wear bright colors and patterns.
No matter what your body type is, always wear clothes that make you feel comfortable and confident.

ACCESSORIZING

When it comes to accessorizing, there are a few things to keep in mind.
The first thing to consider is what you're going to wear the accessory with. For example, if you're going to wear a necklace, you'll want to make sure the neckline of your shirt or dress is high enough that the necklace won't be
visible.

The second thing to think about is the type of accessory you're wearing. For example, if you're wearing a necklace, make sure it's not too heavy. If you're wearing a bracelet, make sure it's not too tight.

The third thing to consider is the color of the accessory. For example, if you're wearing a green shirt, you might not want to wear a green necklace. The same goes for shoes and handbags.

The fourth thing to consider is the style of the accessory. For example, if you're wearing a big, chunky necklace, you might not want to wear a big, chunky bracelet. If you're wearing a small, dainty necklace, you might not want to wear a big, dainty bracelet.

The fifth thing to consider is the occasion. For example, if you're going to a formal event, you might want to wear a formal dress and formal accessories. If you're going to a casual event, you might want to wear a casual dress and casual accessories.

CREATING A NEW LOOK

After a few seasons of wearing the same clothes, I was getting a bit bored of my style. I wanted to try something new, but didn't know how to go about it. A friend of mine recommended I go to a styling session with a personal shopper.

I wasn't sure if it was the right thing for me, but I decided to give it a try. The session was really helpful. The personal shopper showed me how to put together outfits that I never would have thought of on my own. I left with a whole new look and felt much more confident.

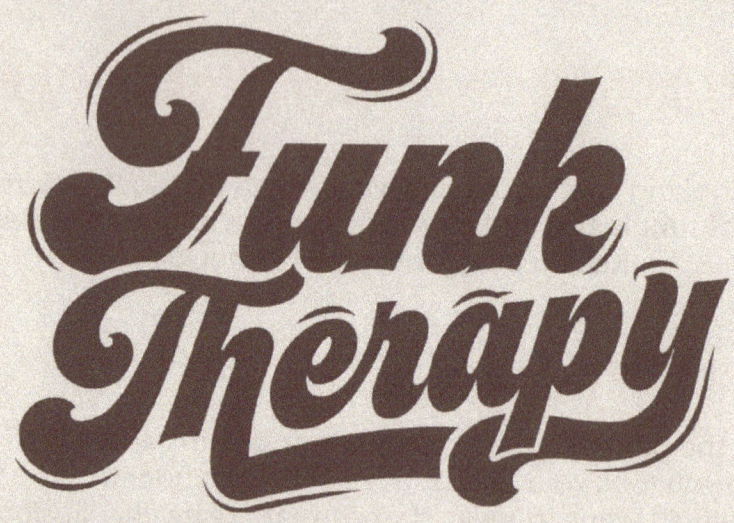

Funk Therapy

Funky	Trendy	Cool	Hip

Wear The Music You Love!

Visit our merchandise store on our website:

WWW.FUNKTHERAPYMUSIC.COM

10% Discount code: STAYFUNKY

- Hoodies
- Crop Top
- Sweat Pants
- Bucket Hats
- Slides
- Mugs

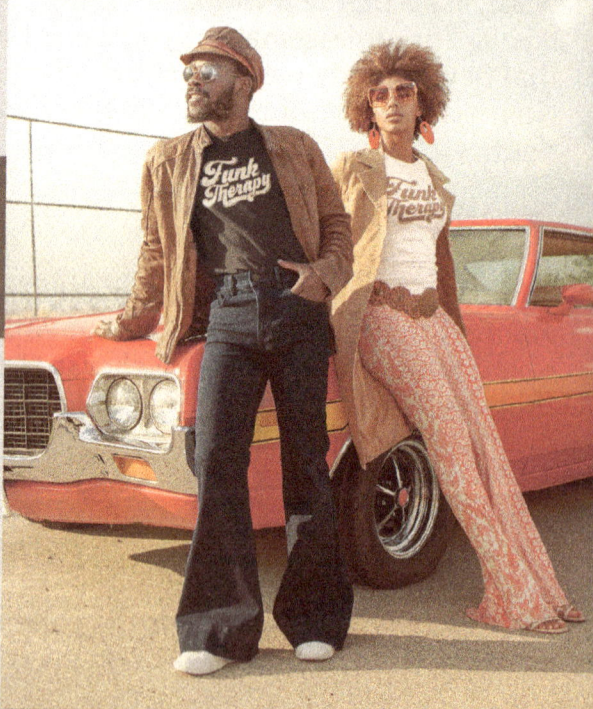

UNISEX T-SHIRTS

Brown T-Shirt

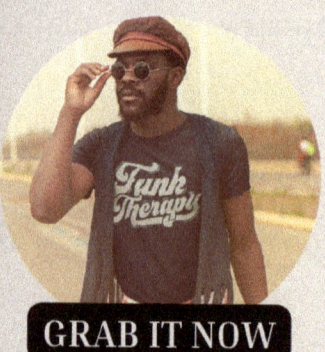

GRAB IT NOW

Orange T-Shirt

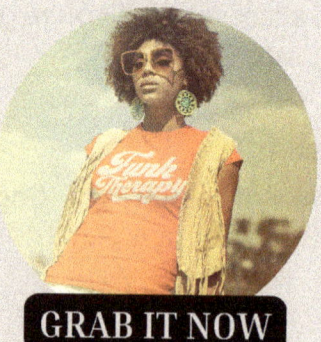

GRAB IT NOW

Beige T-Shirts

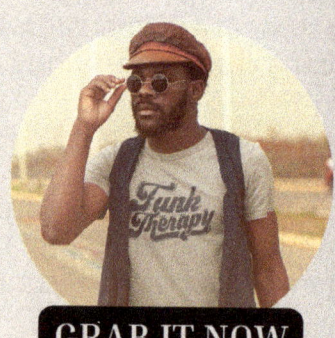

GRAB IT NOW

Join our community
@funktherapy2

THE TOP NATURAL ANTI WRINKLES FIGHTERS

As we age, our skin begins to show signs of wear and tear. wrinkles, fine lines, and age spots are all common skin problems that can make us look older than we really are.
While there are many cosmetic products available to help reduce the appearance of wrinkles, many of these products contain harsh chemicals that can be harmful to our skin.
thankfully, there are many natural products that can help reduce the appearance of wrinkles without the use of harsh chemicals. Here are eight of the best:

WHAT ARE THE BENEFITS OF USING NATURAL PRODUCTS TO REDUCE WRINKLES?

There are many benefits to using natural products to reduce wrinkles. Some of the most notable benefits include:

1. INCREASED COLLAGEN PRODUCTION

One of the main benefits of using natural products to reduce wrinkles is that they can help to increase collagen production. Collagen is responsible for keeping skin looking smooth and elastic, so increased collagen production can help to reduce the appearance of wrinkles.

2. MOISTURE RETENTION

Another benefit of using natural products is that they can help to retain moisture in the skin. This is important because moisture helps to keep skin looking healthy and youthful.

3. ANTIOXIDANTS -

Natural products also often contain antioxidants, which can help to protect the skin from free radicals. Free radicals can damage the skin and lead to the formation of wrinkles.
All of these are important benefits that can help to reduce the appearance of wrinkles.

THE TOP ANTI-AGING PRODUCTS OUT THERE

1. Coconut oil.
This wonder oil has anti-inflammatory and anti-bacterial properties that can help reduce the appearance of wrinkles. It can also help to moisturize and protect your skin against environmental damage.

2. Aloe vera.
This plant is a natural skin healer that can help to reduce the appearance of wrinkles and fine lines. It is also packed with antioxidants that can help protect your skin against free radical damage.

3. Rosehip oil.
This oil is rich in vitamins A and C, which are both important for fighting wrinkles. Rosehip oil can also help to improve skin elasticity and hydration.

4. Pomegranate seed oil.
This oil is a powerful antioxidant that can help to protect your skin against free radical damage. It can also help to stimulate collagen production, which can help reduce the appearance of wrinkles.

5. Black seed oil.
This oil is rich in essential fatty acids and antioxidants, both of which are important for fighting wrinkles. Black seed oil can also help to improve skin elasticity and tone.

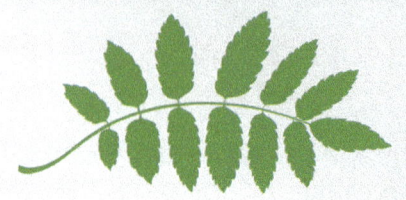

WEST END ORGANIX

Ageless Beauty, Organic Health

BLACK SEED OIL

HEALTHY IMMUNE SYSTEM
INFLAMMATORY RESPONSE

www.westendorganix.com

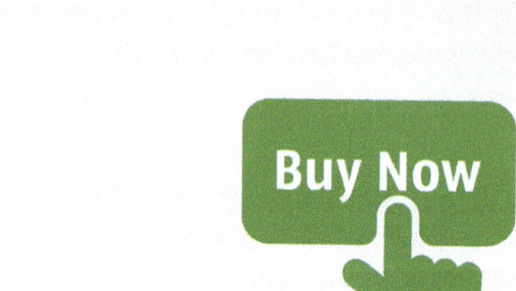

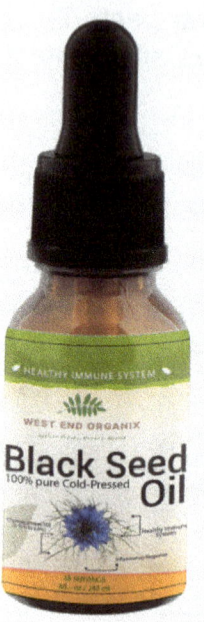

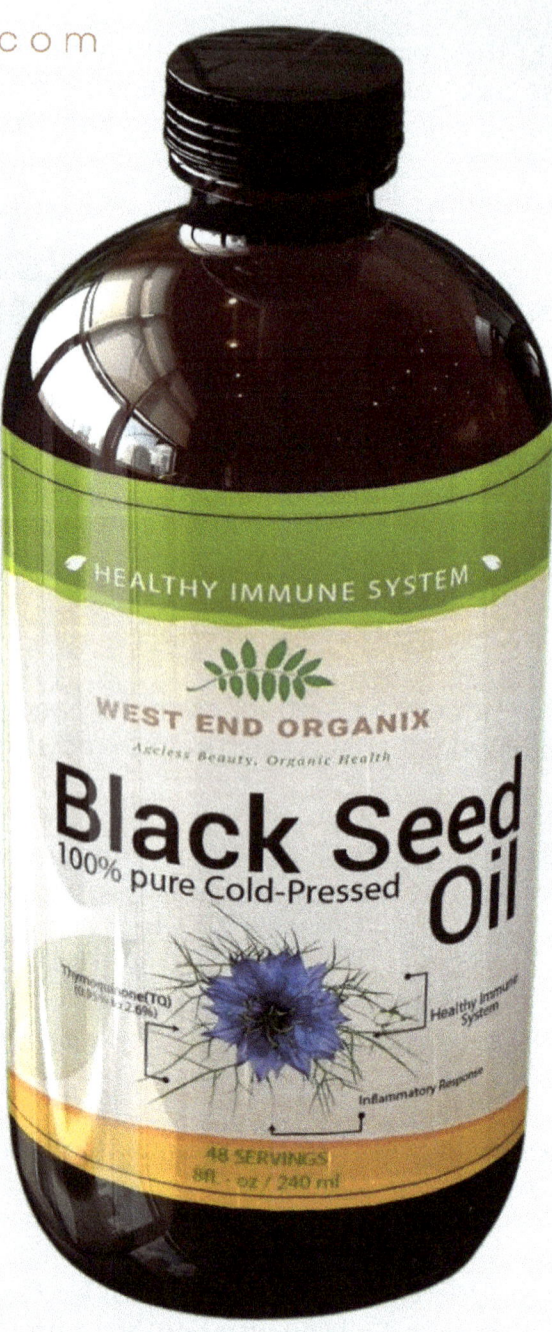

HOW TO GET FIT IN 2023!
NO MORE EXCUSES!

There are a few things you should keep in mind when setting fitness goals for 2023. First, make sure your goals are realistic and achievable. You don't want to set yourself up for disappointment by aiming too high. Second, make sure your goals are specific. Saying you want to be "fit" is too vague, but saying you want to be able to run a marathon in six months is much more manageable. Finally, make sure your goals are time-based.
Having a deadline will help keep you motivated and on track.

HOW TO CREATE A WORKOUT ROUTINE THAT FITS YOUR LIFESTYLE

Creating a workout routine that fits your lifestyle can be difficult, but it's not impossible. You'll need to find a time that works for you, create a routine that is challenging but not too difficult, and make sure to stick to it! Here are a few tips to help you get started.

First, find a time that works for you. Whether you want to workout in the morning, in the evening, or on the weekends, find a time that you will be able to stick to. If you're not a morning person, don't try to workout in the morning. Find a time that works for your schedule and your body.

Second, create a routine that is challenging but not too difficult. If your routine is too difficult, you're more likely to skip workouts. On the other hand, if your routine is too easy, you won't see results. Find a routine that is the right level of difficulty for you and that you can stick to.

Finally, make sure to stick to your routine! Creating a workout routine is the first step, but sticking to it is just as important. If you find yourself struggling to stick to your routine, ask a friend to join you or find a workout buddy. Having someone to workout with will help you stay on track.

HOW TO EAT HEALTHY AND STAY MOTIVATED

There are many different ways to eat healthy and stay motivated. Some people like to have a set routine, while others prefer to change things up every day.
Here are a few tips to help you get started:

1. Start by making small changes.
If you try to overhaul your entire diet all at once, you're likely to get overwhelmed and give up. Start by making small changes, like adding an extra serving of vegetables to your lunch, or swapping out sugary drinks for water.

2. Find healthy recipes that you enjoy.
If you don't enjoy the food you're eating, you're less likely to stick with it. Try searching for healthy recipes online or in cookbooks, and experiment until you find something you really love.

3. Get plenty of protein.
Protein is essential for building muscle and maintaining energy levels. Make sure you're getting enough protein each day by incorporating plenty of high-protein foods into your diet.

4. Stay hydrated.
Drinking plenty of water is essential for good health and can help you stay motivated to eat healthy. Carry a water bottle with you wherever you go, and aim to drink at least eight glasses per day.

5. Take your time.
It's important to eat slowly and savor your food. This will help you feel full sooner and prevent you from overeating.

6. Avoid processed foods
Processed foods are often high in unhealthy fats, sugar, and salt. Avoiding them will help you stay on track with your healthy eating goals.

7. Get moving. Exercise is a great way to stay motivated and healthy. Make sure you're getting enough exercise each week by incorporating regular workouts into your routine.

SLIM & SEXY

Legs, Stretching and warm-up, 25 Squats, 25 Sumo Squats, Repeat, March in place for 20 seconds Stretch muscles, Relax 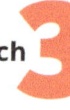 **1**

Abs, Stretching and warm-up, 20 Standing Oblique Twists 30-second Floor Plank, Repeat above, March in place for 20 seconds, Stretch muscles, Relax 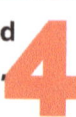 **2**

Arms, Stretching and warm-up, 25 Push-ups, 20 Wall Tricep Pushes, Repeat above, March in place for 20 seconds, Stretch muscles, Relax **3**

Cardio, Stretching and warm-up, 50 Jumping Jacks, 30-second Sprint in place, Repeat above, March in place for 20 seconds, Stretch muscles, Relax 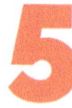 **4**

Combo, Stretching and warm-up, 10 Squats & 10 Sumo Squats, 10 Standing Oblique Twists, March in place for 20 seconds, 20 Push-ups, 25 Jumping Jacks, March in place for 20 seconds, Stretch muscles, Relax **5**

Choose from Day 1-4 to work on your chosen area: Legs, Abs, Arms, or Cardio" **6**

Rest!

Take a break! You deserve it. **7**

TWO WEEKS PROGRAM

Body & Mind Self-care Exercise

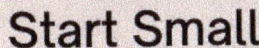

Start Small

You can start from small goals to big ones, from just a simple walk day to a full spa-day. Your choice!

 **Start to set boundaries**

 **Make a daily routine steps**

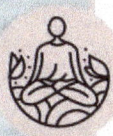 **Go Meditate**

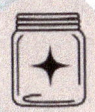 **Keep & write a gratitude jar**

 **Tidy up your space**

Reminder

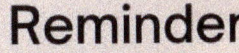

It can be a long journey, but in the end will always be worth it.

Korey Fitzgerald

**PROFESSIONAL HOLLYWOOD
HAIR STYLIST AND BARBER**

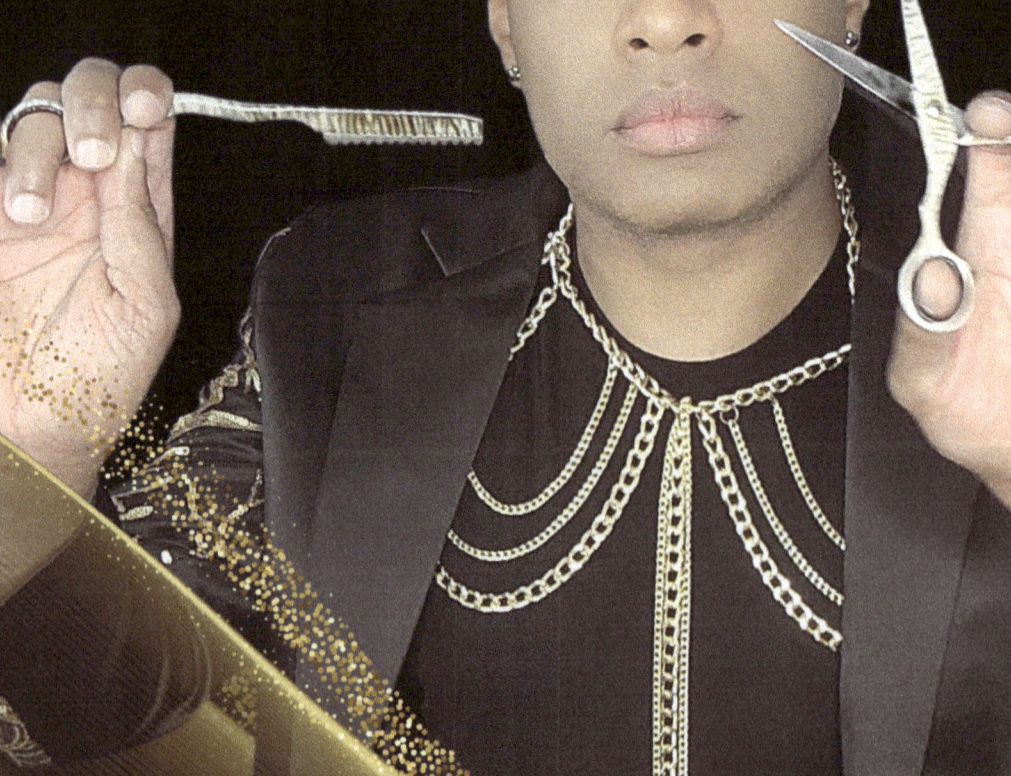

CONTACT

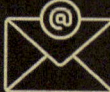 KOREYCFITZ@GMAIL.COM

 @HOLLYWOODHAIRKING

STRATEGIES TO GET
YOUR MUSIC HEARD BY MORE PEOPLE!

1. DEVELOP A STRONG ONLINE PRESENCE.

 In order to develop a strong online presence, it is important to first identify your target audience. Once you know your target audience, you can focus your marketing efforts on reaching them where they are spending the majority of their time online. Additionally, it is important to keep your website and social media profiles up-to-date and consistent with your branding. By doing so, you will create a strong online presence that helps you reach your target audience and grow your business.

2. USE SOCIAL MEDIA TO MARKET YOUR MUSIC.

There are many different ways to use social media to market your music. You can create a profile on music-specific sites like SoundCloud or Bandcamp, or general sites like Facebook or Twitter. You can also create a YouTube channel to share your music videos.
Once you have created a profile, you can start sharing your music with your friends and followers. Make sure to post about upcoming shows, release dates, and other news related to your music. You can also use social media to connect with other musicians and fans.
Social media is a great way to connect with your fans and promote your music. Make sure to use it to your advantage!

3. MARKET YOUR MUSIC TO RADIO STATIONS.

 When it comes to marketing your music, radio stations can be a great way to get your music out there. However, it's important to remember that not all radio stations are created equal. There are a few things you need to keep in mind when targeting radio stations.

First, you'll want to make sure your music is radio-friendly. That means it needs to be well-produced and have a strong hook. Radio stations are typically looking for music that will get people's attention and keep them listening.

Second, you'll need to research the right radio stations to target. Not all stations are interested in all genres of music. Make sure you target stations that are a good fit for your music.

Finally, be prepared to do some work to get your music played on the air. Most radio stations won't just play your music without some kind of push from you. You'll need to reach out to the right people at the station and make a good case for why your music should be played.

If you can follow these tips, you'll be well on your way to getting your music heard on the radio.

4. PLAY LIVE SHOWS.

 Play live shows. Play live shows as much as possible. The more shows you play, the more people will know about your music, and the better you will get at performing.
Plus, playing live shows is a great way to get your music out there and make connections in the music industry.

By using these strategies, you can make sure that more people hear your music and appreciate your talent.

YOUR MUSIC CONSULTANT

"You Believe And So Do We"

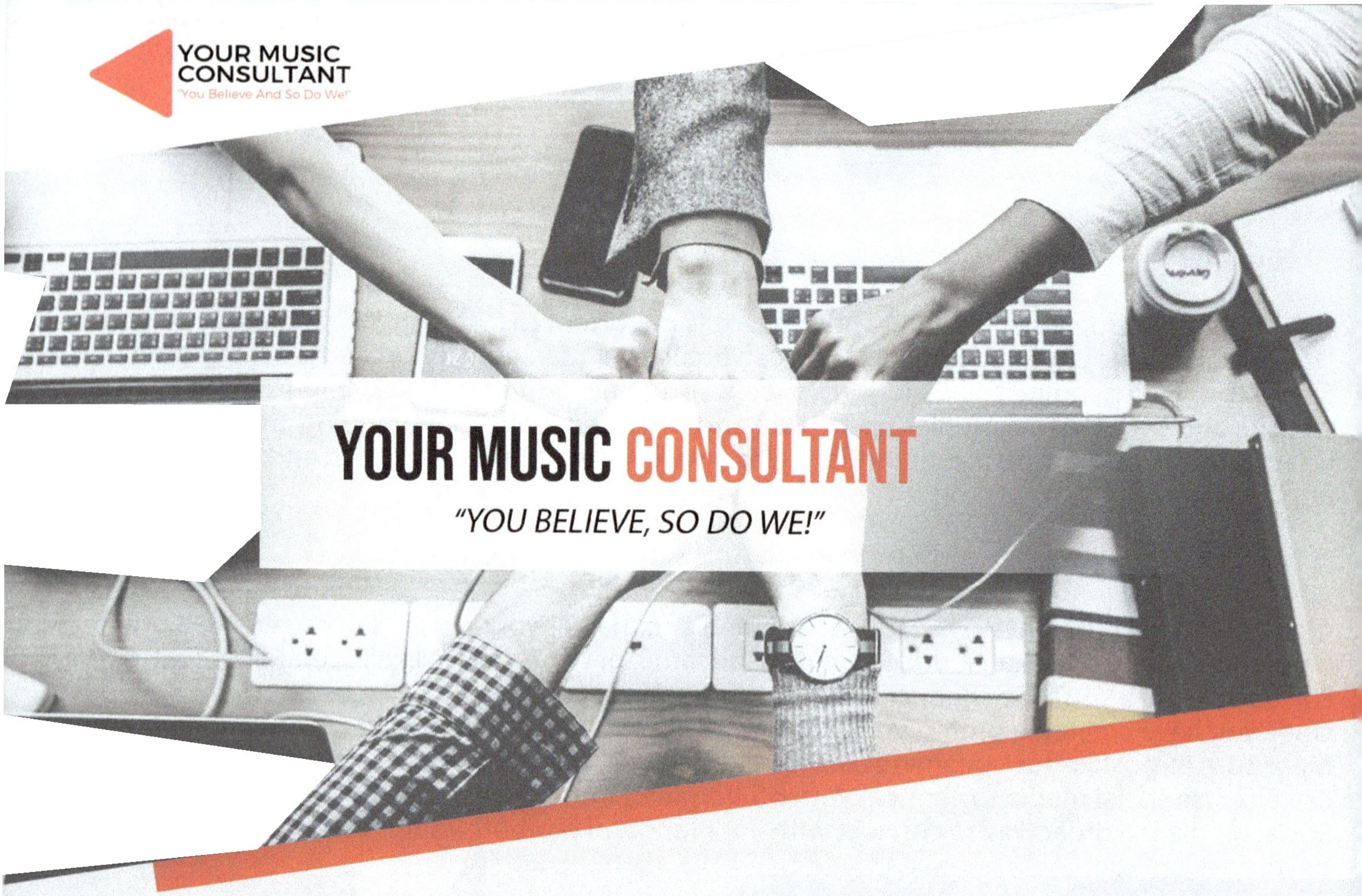

YOUR MUSIC CONSULTANT

"YOU BELIEVE, SO DO WE!"

We Can Help You To Grow Your Business

We are a monthly based service, we put faith in artists who has major potential, believed in them, and who are willing to spend their time and own money to work with us in building a successful music career!

Digital Marketing Services

SOCIAL MEDIA - STREAMING SERVICES - MUSIC DISTRIBUTION - PRESS RELEASE - PRESS DISTRIBUTION - PR

Radio Airplay and TV Commercial

TERRESTRIAL AND DIGITAL RADIO CAMPAIGN AL GENRES EXCEPT HEAVY METAL - CABLE TV AND MAJOR NETWORK COMMERCIAL

Licensing & Booking

CONCERTS, LIVE MUSIC, EVENTS, CLUB NIGHTS - RED CARPETS - FOREIGN LICENSING AND SUBOPUBLISHING

Why Choose Us ?

3 DECADES OF MUSIC BUSINESS EXPERIENCE
Platinium and Gold Records

MOTOWN RECORDS
UNIVERSAL
SONY
CAPITOL RECORDS

WE WORKED WITH:
Kanye West - Jay Z - Stevie Wonder - Michael Jackson - Germaine Jackson Smokey Robinson - Dionne Warwick - Cheryl Lynn - The Originals -

📞 **1 -818-514-0038**
(Ext. 1)
Monday - Friday / 9am to 6pm

FIND US :

www.YourMusicConsultant.com
30721 Russell Ranch Road Suite 140 Westlake Village, USA
Email : info@yourmusicconsultant.com

OSCAR WORTHY MOVIES

1. EVERYTHING EVERYWHERE ALL AT ONCE

There are no amount of words that can describe the conventional breaker hit of the year, that made us feel the thrust of raw and experimental cinema. Michelle Yeoh's mind-bending performance itself deserves a separate nomination for making us root for the most badass action role in recent times. You can stream it on Hulu.

2. THE FABLEMANS

Going by the decorated track record of Steven Spielberg and the magnificent film itself, The Fablemans is one of the strongest movies of the year with a perfect chance of landing that OSCARS nomination. I can't help but remember that quote by Bong Joon-Ho at the 92nd Academy Awards (which in turn was a Martin Scorcese reference), The most Personal is the most Creative.

Regarded as one of the most intimate works of the director, the film works like a semi-biographical ode to his childhood fascination for movies. You can still catch it on the big screen.

3.THE WHALE

If there was a combination of words for "most hyped" and a "grand return", then it would simply be The Whale. I don't want to take anything away from the critic's darling of the year and silently root for Brendan Fraser to receive his much-deserved nomination (God I hope I don't Jinx it). And also wish that the Academy voters ignore the minute flaws (subjective), and advance the feature for the award season.

That being said, we have seen such festival favourite films getting snubbed more than often, and maybe it will be a good thing no attach all my emotions to this one.

4. TÁR

Perhaps, there is no argument about Cate Blanchett's name inside the Best Actress envelope card (Yes, I am that sure). Along with the feature film's fair share of nominations this season. Based on the true story of a musician's rise and fall, the electrifying film is not only a goosebumps raiser but also a cinematic achievement.

It is also the only movie on this list, for which I can give a personal guarantee (obviously with terms and conditions) of a pretty fine trajectory at the Academy Awards. I guess you'll have to wait a bit longer for its streaming destination.

5. RRR

Believe me, when I say that I have zero personal bias here. If you have, by any chance, followed the award season buzz this year, then you might be aware of the fandom that RRR has created among professional critics. The sheer amount of passion with which the western cine-goers have praised the movie is almost in the same volume as the Desi cheer.

It can not only end India's dry run at the OSCARS but also drench us in a couple of golden trophies this year. Perhpas, RRR is our strongest contender after Shaunak Sen's magnificent documentary All That Breathes. You can stream the historical epic on Netflix.

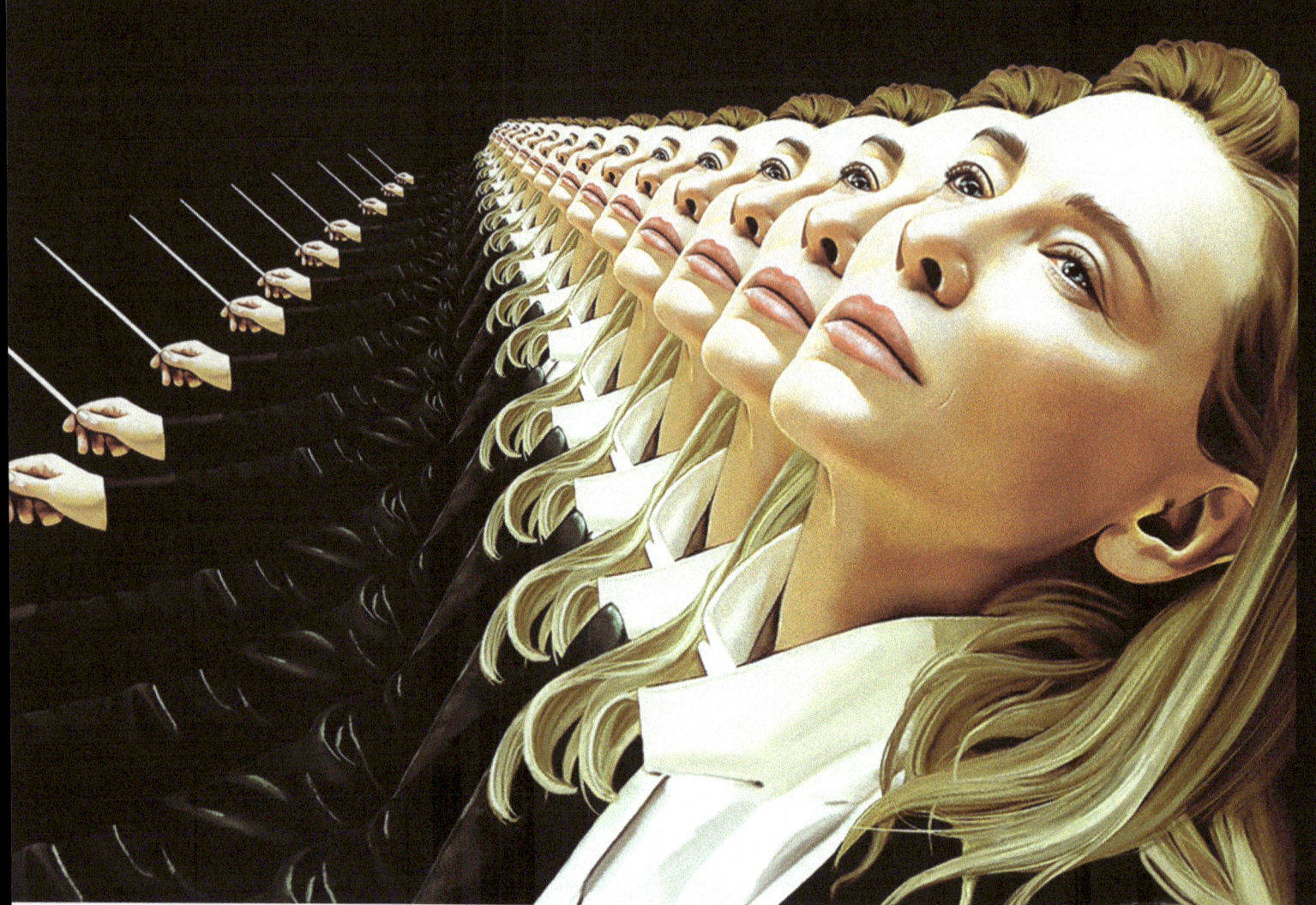

HOW CAN YOU HELP STOP
HUMAN TRAFFICKING

Anyone can join in the fight against human trafficking. Here are a few ideas to consider.

Learn the indicators of human trafficking on the TIP Office's website or by taking a training. Human trafficking awareness training is available for individuals, businesses, first responders, law enforcement, educators, and federal employees, among others.
If you are in the United States and believe someone may be a victim of human trafficking, call the 24-hour National Human Trafficking Hotline at 1-888-373-7888 or report an emergency to law enforcement by calling 911. Trafficking victims, whether or not U.S. citizens, are eligible for services and immigration assistance.

Volunteer and support anti-trafficking efforts in your community .
Meet with and/or write to your local, state, and federal elected officials to let them know you care about combating human trafficking and ask what they are doing to address it.
Be well-informed. Set up a web alert to receive current human trafficking news.
Also, check out CNN's Freedom Project for more stories on the different forms of human trafficking around the world.

Host an awareness-raising event to watch and discuss films about human trafficking.
For example, learn how modern slavery exists today; watch an investigative documentary about sex trafficking; or discover how forced labor can affect global food supply chains. Alternatively, contact your local library and ask for assistance identifying an appropriate book and ask them to host the event.

Organize a fundraiser and donate the proceeds to an anti-trafficking organization .
Encourage your local schools or school district to include human trafficking in their curricula and to develop protocols for identifying and reporting a suspected case of human trafficking or responding to a potential victim.

Use your social media platforms to raise awareness about human trafficking, using the following hashtags: #endtrafficking, #freedomfirst.
Think about whether your workplace is trauma-informed and reach out to management or the Human Resources team to urge implementation of trauma-informed business practices .

Become a mentor to a young person or someone in need.
Traffickers often target people who are going through a difficult time or who lack strong support systems. As a mentor, you can be involved in new and positive experiences in that person's life during a formative time.

Parents and Caregivers: Learn how human traffickers often target and recruit youth
and who to turn to for help in potentially dangerous situations. Host community conversations with parent teacher associations, law enforcement, schools, and community members regarding safeguarding children in your community.
Youth: Learn how to recognize traffickers' recruitment tactics , how to safely navigate out of a suspicious or uncomfortable situations, and how to reach out for help at any time.
Faith-Based Communities : Host awareness events and community forums with anti-trafficking leaders or collectively support a local victim service provider.
Businesses: Provide jobs, internships, skills training, and other opportunities to trafficking survivors.
Take steps to investigate and prevent trafficking in your supply chains by consulting the Responsible Sourcing Tool and Comply Chain to develop effective management systems to detect, prevent, and combat human trafficking.
College Students: Take action on your campus.

Editions L.A.

DIGITAL CREATIVE AGENCY

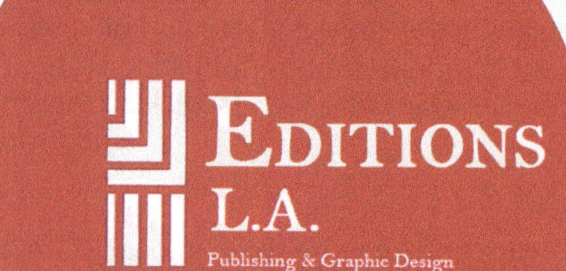

We Transform Your Vision Into Creative Results

Editions L.A. is a full-service agency based in Los Angeles. Our company is a collective of amazing people striving to build delightful services
We believe that is all about getting your message across clearly and with a "Wow!" thrown in for good measure.

Our Awesome Services

Branding

We build, style and tone your brand identity from the ground up.
We rebrand established bands, brands or businesses.

Merchandise Store
Website design and E-Commerce
Website updates

Digital Marketing

CD Cover | Banners | Logo design | Flyers | Brochures | Leaflets | Print ads | Magazine covers & artworks
Facebook / twitter / instagram / youtube artworks | Book cover
Infographics | Icon Design |
| TshirtsProduct Labels | Presentation slides
Corporate graphics
Professional photo editing & enhancing
Redesign existing elements
YouTube Optimization and Monetization
Youtube Video Editing
Lyric Video and Advertising Design.

Publishing

BOOK COVER DESIGN
EBOOK FORMATTING SERVICES
and distribution on major platforms
(Amazon, Barnes & Nobles..)

Tell us about your dream and we will make it true!

Editions L.A.
7210 Jordan Avenue Suite B42, Canoga Park, California 91303, United States
info@edtions-la.com
Website: www.editions-la.com

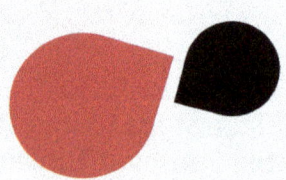

HOW CAN YOU HELP STOP
HUMAN TRAFFICKING

LEARN THE RED FLAGS

Human Trafficking Indicators
While not an exhaustive list, these are some key red flags that could alert you
to a potential trafficking situation that should be reported:

Living with employer
Poor living conditions
Multiple people in cramped space
Inability to speak to individual alone
Answers appear to be scripted and rehearsed
Employer is holding identity documents
Signs of physical abuse
Submissive or fearful
Unpaid or paid very little
Under 18 and in prostitution

QUESTIONS TO ASK

Assuming you have the opportunity to speak with a potential victim privately and without jeop-
ardizing the victim's safety because the trafficker is watching,
here are some sample questions to ask to follow up on the red flags you became alert to:

Can you leave your job if you want to?
Can you come and go as you please?
Have you been hurt or threatened if you tried to leave?
Has your family been threatened?
Do you live with your employer?
Where do you sleep and eat?
Are you in debt to your employer?
Do you have your passport/identification? Who has it?

WHERE TO GET HELP

If you believe you have identified someone still in the trafficking situation, alert law enforcement
immediately at the numbers provided below. It may be unsafe to attempt to rescue a trafficking
victim. You have no way of knowing how the trafficker may react and retaliate against the victim
and you. If, however, you identify a victim who has escaped the trafficking situation, there are a
number of organizations to whom the victim could be referred for help with shelter, medical care,
legal assistance, and other critical services. In this case, call the National Human Trafficking Hotline
described below.

911 EMERGENCY

For urgent situations, notify local law enforcement immediately by calling 911. You may also want
to alert the National Human Trafficking Hotline described below so that they can ensure response
by law enforcement officials knowledgeable about human trafficking.

1-888-373-7888 National Human Trafficking Hotline

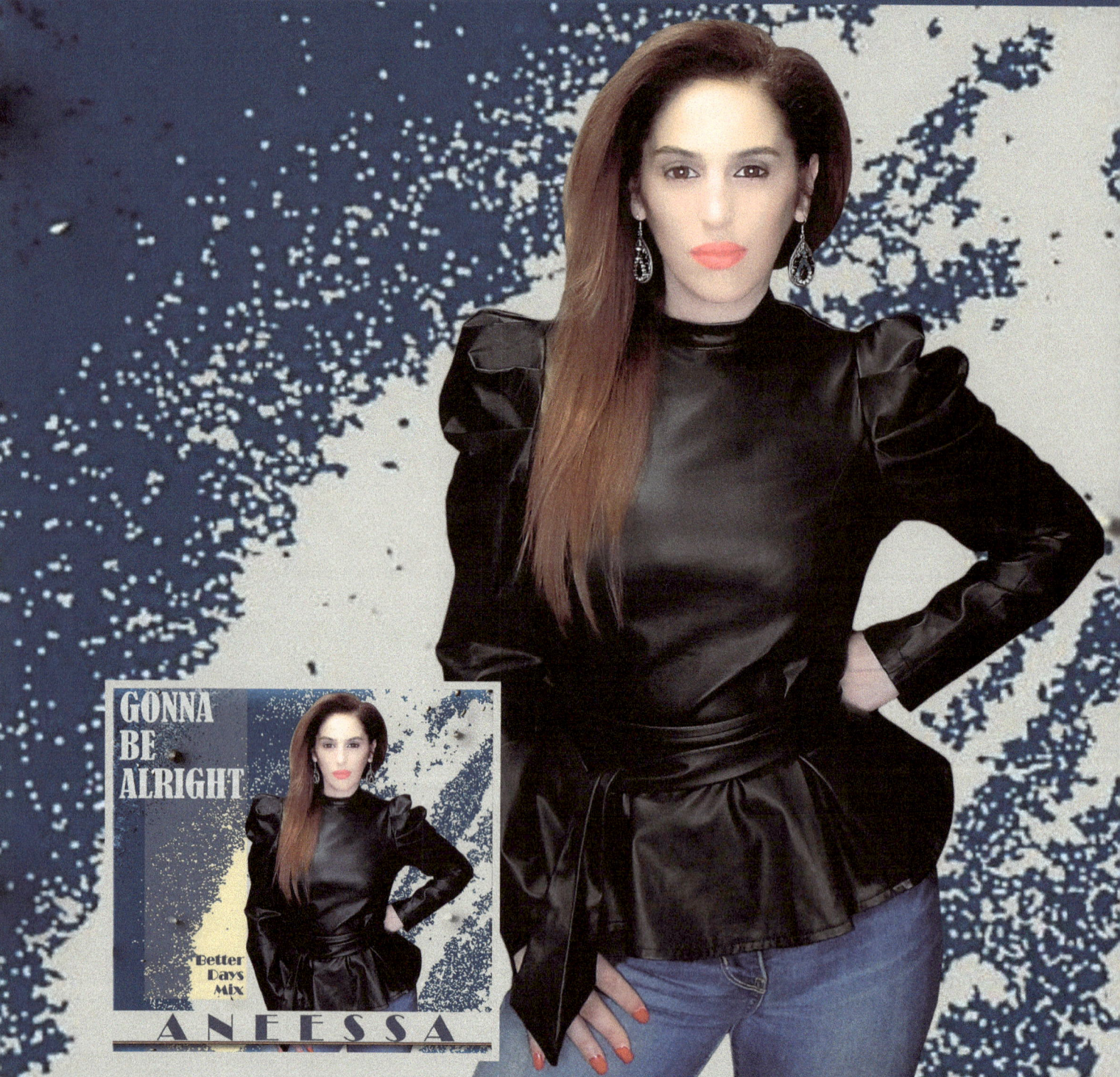

Lightning Source UK Ltd.
Milton Keynes UK
UKHW051812270123
415999UK00012B/29